TABLE OF CONTENTS

I0408674

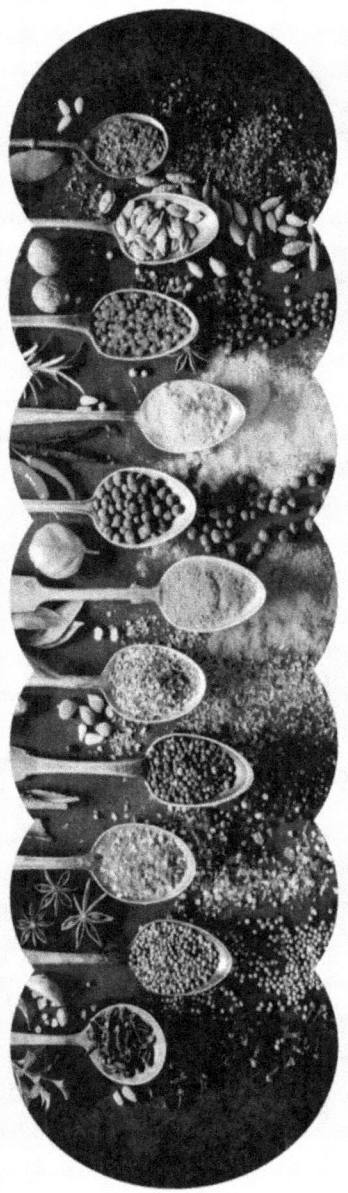

Introduction:

Welcome to "Pawsitive Balance: Exploring Holistic Health for Dogs and Cats." In this comprehensive guide, we embark on a journey towards nurturing the well-being of our beloved four-legged companions using a natural and holistic approach to health and healing. As we delve into the world of holistic pet care, it is crucial to understand the unique anatomical differences between cats and dogs and the sensitivity of a cat's digestive system.

Our feline friends, with their mysterious charm, are captivating creatures with distinctive dietary requirements. Cats are obligate carnivores, meaning their bodies are specifically adapted to thrive on a diet primarily composed of meat. Their digestive systems are designed to efficiently break down and utilize proteins, making them highly dependent on vital amino acids like taurine and arachidonic acid, which are essential for their overall health and well-being.

Due to the sensitivity of a cat's digestive system, even completely natural ingredients, such as herbs, spices, and essential oils, may not be suitable for them. Unlike dogs, cats lack certain liver enzymes, which hinders their ability to metabolize certain compounds found in plants and herbs. Consequently, some seemingly innocuous ingredients that benefit dogs can pose risks to our feline companions.

In "Pawsitive Balance," we have taken utmost care to ensure that every recipe and ingredient is meticulously researched and tailored to the specific nutritional requirements of both cats and dogs. The recipes provided have been crafted with a deep understanding of their distinct anatomies, ensuring that each ingredient serves a purpose in promoting their optimal health.

However, it is essential to remember that the recipes containing herbs, spices, and essential oils are exclusively intended for dogs, as they have a more versatile digestive system that can tolerate these ingredients. For the well-being of our feline friends, we have specially curated recipes that adhere to their unique dietary needs, avoiding any potentially harmful substances.

Rest assured that the ingredients used in this book are backed by scientific research, and the recipes have been tested to ensure their safety and efficacy for our furry companions. The holistic approach offered in "Pawsitive Balance" seeks to provide a balanced and nourishing diet while respecting the sensitivities of our beloved cats.

As we explore the realm of holistic health for dogs and cats, it is crucial to remember that these recipes are meant to complement traditional veterinary care. If you have any doubts or concerns about your pet's dietary needs or the suitability of specific ingredients, always consult with a qualified professional. Your veterinarian will be an invaluable partner in tailoring a holistic health plan that caters to your pets' unique requirements.

With "Pawsitive Balance" as your guide, let us embark on this fulfilling journey towards providing our cherished pets with the love, care, and holistic support they deserve. May this book be a beacon of knowledge and compassion, strengthening the bond we share with our furry companions as we work together to create a happier and healthier life for them.

Chapter 1. Understanding the Holistic Approach to Treating and Healing

Embracing a natural holistic approach to treating and healing your pets' common ailments offers a myriad of benefits compared to relying solely on pharmacy medicine. This approach acknowledges the innate healing power of the body and focuses on addressing the root cause of issues rather than just suppressing symptoms. Let's explore some of the advantages of choosing a natural holistic approach for your pets' well-being:

1. Gentle and Non-Toxic: Natural remedies often use plant-based ingredients and gentle methods that are less likely to cause adverse reactions or side effects in pets. They are safer and less harsh on their systems, making them suitable for long-term use without compromising their overall health.

2. Whole-Body Healing: Holistic treatments take into account the interconnectedness of the body, mind, and spirit. By addressing all aspects of your pet's well-being, these therapies support holistic healing, promoting overall balance and wellness.

3. Prevention-Oriented: Natural holistic care focuses on preventing health issues before they arise. By adopting preventive measures, such as a balanced diet, regular exercise, and stress reduction techniques, you can proactively support your pet's health, reducing the likelihood of future ailments.

4. Reduced Dependency on Medications: Traditional pharmacy medicine often relies on medications that may only provide temporary relief for specific symptoms. A natural holistic approach seeks to eliminate or minimize the use of pharmaceuticals, thus reducing the risk of adverse effects and drug interactions.

5. Individualized Care: Holistic treatments are tailored to your pet's unique needs, taking into account their specific health conditions and temperament. This personalized approach ensures that your pet receives the most suitable and effective care possible.

6. Emphasis on Well-Being: Holistic care goes beyond treating physical ailments; it also addresses emotional and behavioral issues. By focusing on emotional well-being, it helps pets feel happier and more content, leading to a higher quality of life.

7. Complementary to Conventional Care: Natural holistic approaches can be used alongside conventional veterinary medicine. Integrating both approaches allows for a comprehensive and balanced approach to your pet's health, maximizing their chances of recovery.

8. Environmental Consciousness: Many natural remedies and holistic practices use sustainable and eco-friendly ingredients and methods, making them better for the environment and reducing the ecological footprint of pet care.

9. Empowerment as a Pet Owner: Adopting a natural holistic approach empowers you as a pet owner to actively participate in your pet's care and well-being. It encourages you to be proactive in managing their health and forming a deeper bond with them.

10. Long-Term Health Benefits: By promoting overall health and wellness, a natural holistic approach can lead to improved longevity and a better quality of life for your pets, ensuring they live happy, healthy, and fulfilling lives.

Incorporating natural holistic approaches into your pets' lives can lead to a harmonious and holistic journey towards their well-being. It fosters a deeper understanding of their needs and empowers you to be a proactive and loving advocate for their health. By embracing this natural path, you can nurture a stronger connection with your pets and provide them with a life filled with vitality and joy.

Choosing a natural approach to healing your pets' ailments can often be less costly compared to relying solely on traditional pharmacy medicine. Natural remedies and herbal treatments are readily available for purchase online and are easy to access, making them a cost-effective and convenient option for pet owners. Here are some key points to consider:

1. Affordability of Natural Remedies: Natural remedies, including herbal treatments, are often more affordable than prescription medications. Traditional pharmacy medicine can be costly, especially for long-term treatments or chronic conditions. In contrast, natural remedies can offer a cost-effective alternative without compromising on effectiveness.

2. Reduced Veterinary Visits: By proactively addressing your pets' health with natural remedies, you may be able to reduce the frequency of veterinary visits. Preventive measures and holistic care can help keep your pets healthier, minimizing the need for expensive medical treatments.

3. DIY Options: Many natural remedies can be prepared at home with simple ingredients, further reducing costs. DIY treatments allow you to tailor remedies to your pets' specific needs, making it a budget-friendly and customizable approach.

4. Access to Herbal Remedies Online: The internet offers a wealth of resources where you can find and purchase herbal remedies for pets. Numerous reputable online retailers specialize in natural pet products, providing a convenient way to access a wide range of herbal remedies.

5. Availability of Information: With the internet at your fingertips, you can easily find information and resources on natural healing for pets. Reputable websites, articles, and forums offer insights into various herbal remedies and holistic practices.

6. Fewer Side Effects: Natural remedies often have fewer side effects compared to pharmaceutical medications. This can translate to fewer unexpected expenses related to managing adverse reactions or seeking additional treatments.

7. Long-Term Savings: Investing in your pets' long-term well-being through a natural approach can lead to potential savings on future medical expenses. Preventive care and maintaining their overall health can help avoid costly medical interventions down the road.

8. Holistic Wellness Benefits: Natural remedies support overall holistic wellness, which can positively impact multiple aspects of your pets' health. Improved well-being may lead to reduced health issues, saving you money on medical treatments.

9. Customization for Individual Needs: Herbal remedies can be tailored to suit your pets' specific health concerns. This customization ensures that you are addressing their unique needs, potentially leading to more targeted and effective healing.

10. Complementary to Conventional Medicine: A natural approach can work in harmony with traditional veterinary care. Integrating both methods allows you to provide comprehensive care for your pets while potentially minimizing the need for expensive treatments.

By embracing a natural approach to healing your pets' ailments, you can not only save on costs but also enhance their overall well-being. Herbal remedies and holistic practices offer a budget-friendly, accessible, and effective way to support your pets' health and happiness. As a responsible and caring pet owner, exploring natural alternatives can lead to a fulfilling and satisfying journey in providing the best care for your furry companions.

As you explore the benefits of a natural approach to healing your pets' ailments, I invite you to visit my website, craftycomeupsandmore.bigcartel.com, where you can find a selection of holistic pet care products from my brand EK Cosmetics that have been crafted with love and care. My website offers a range of handcrafted remedies, salves, ointments, and more, all made from natural ingredients that prioritize the well-being of your furry companions.

By choosing products from Crafty Comeups and More, you are embracing a holistic journey towards your pets' health and happiness. Each item is carefully formulated to provide gentle and effective relief, promoting their overall wellness while being mindful of their physical, emotional, and spiritual needs.

You'll discover that these holistic pet care products complement the natural approach to healing, empowering you to provide the best care for your pets in the comfort of your home. From soothing salves for itchy paws to herbal remedies for common ailments, my offerings are designed to support your pets' health in a safe and nurturing manner.

By visiting craftycomeupsandmore.bigcartel.com, you'll have the opportunity to explore a variety of options that align with your pets' unique requirements. Each product is made with quality natural ingredients, and their efficacy is backed by research and a commitment to excellence.

As you embark on this journey towards holistic pet care, I am honored to share my passion for providing safe, non-toxic, and effective solutions for your furry friends. Your pets deserve the best, and Crafty Comeups and More is here to assist you in nurturing their well-being through the power of nature.

Thank you for considering Crafty Comeups and More as your go-to resource for holistic pet care products. I am thrilled to be part of your pets' health and happiness journey. Together, we can create a harmonious and holistic environment where your beloved companions thrive in vitality and joy. Visit craftycomeupsandmore.bigcartel.com today to explore our offerings and take the next step in providing the best for your pets' well-being.

Pets are not just animals; they are cherished members of our families, and their well-being goes beyond their physical health. Emphasizing the wholeness of pets involves acknowledging and nurturing their physical, emotional, and spiritual aspects. Understanding and addressing these interconnected elements are key to providing holistic care that fosters a happy and balanced life for our beloved companions.

1. The Physical Aspect:
Pets' physical well-being is the foundation of their overall health. This includes their diet, exercise, and proper medical care. Providing a nutritious and balanced diet tailored to their individual needs supports their immune system, energy levels, and organ function. Regular exercise is vital to keep them physically fit and mentally stimulated, promoting a sense of vitality and joy. Ensuring they receive regular veterinary check-ups and preventive care safeguards against potential health issues, setting the stage for a healthier life.

2. The Emotional Aspect:
   Pets experience a vast range of emotions, just like humans. They can feel joy, love, fear, and stress. Acknowledging their emotional aspect means being attuned to their feelings and understanding their behavioral cues. Creating a nurturing and loving environment, filled with affection and positive interactions, fosters emotional well-being. Pets thrive on companionship and feel a sense of security when they are part of a caring family. Being present for them during challenging times, such as illness or change, helps strengthen their emotional resilience.

3. The Spiritual Aspect:

The spiritual connection between pets and their humans is profound and goes beyond physical presence. It is a bond of unconditional love, trust, and loyalty. Embracing the spiritual aspect means recognizing the unique and meaningful role pets play in our lives. They offer companionship and a sense of purpose, enriching our existence. Nurturing this spiritual connection involves being present and mindful in our interactions, creating moments of shared joy and tranquility.

Recognizing the wholeness of pets means treating them as sentient beings with multifaceted needs. By addressing their physical, emotional, and spiritual aspects, we create a harmonious and balanced environment for them to flourish. As responsible pet owners, we have the privilege and responsibility to provide comprehensive care that embraces all aspects of their being.

Our pets bring us immeasurable joy, unconditional love, and invaluable life lessons. By nurturing their wholeness, we reciprocate this love by ensuring their well-being on every level. This holistic approach is not just about the absence of illness but also about promoting a thriving and fulfilled life for our furry companions. Embracing their wholeness deepens the bond we share with them and enriches our journey together in a profound and meaningful way.

Chapter 2: The Interconnectedness of Body, Mind, and Spirit in Your Pet

As we delve deeper into the world of holistic pet care, it becomes evident that our furry companions are not merely physical beings but intricate beings with interconnected aspects of body, mind, and spirit. Understanding the interplay of these elements is essential in providing comprehensive and nurturing care for our pets.

1. The Body:

The physical aspect of our pets is the most apparent and tangible. Their body is a marvelous biological system, intricately designed to function harmoniously. It is through their body that they experience the world, engaging with their environment, and expressing their emotions. Ensuring their physical well-being involves providing nutritious meals, regular exercise, and proper medical attention. The health of their body forms the foundation for a happy and vibrant life.

2. The Mind:

The emotional and cognitive aspect of our pets is a testament to their intelligence and sensitivity. They experience a wide range of emotions, including joy, fear, anxiety, and contentment. Their minds are attuned to their surroundings, their family members, and other pets, forming connections and bonds that enrich their lives. Understanding their minds involves recognizing their behavioral cues, addressing their emotional needs, and providing a nurturing and stimulating environment. A content and stimulated mind promotes mental well-being and emotional balance.

3. The Spirit:
The spiritual aspect of our pets transcends the physical realm and delves into the realm of unconditional love and profound connections. Their spirit is a source of unwavering loyalty, trust, and compassion. Our pets have an innate ability to provide comfort and companionship during difficult times, offering a sense of solace and support. Nurturing their spirit involves being present with them in moments of joy and sorrow, fostering a deep bond built on trust and affection. This spiritual connection reminds us of the profound impact our pets have on our lives and the interconnectedness we share.

The interplay of body, mind, and spirit in our pets creates a dynamic and holistic existence. The state of one aspect can significantly influence the others, highlighting the importance of a balanced and integrated approach to their care. A healthy body fosters a content mind, while emotional well-being enriches their spirit, forming a harmonious synergy.

As pet owners, embracing the interconnectedness of body, mind, and spirit allows us to provide the best care for our furry companions. By nurturing their physical health, addressing their emotional needs, and cherishing the spiritual bond we share, we create a nurturing and enriching environment for them to thrive.

In the following chapters, we will explore various holistic approaches and natural remedies that cater to the interconnected well-being of our pets. By incorporating these practices into their lives, we can deepen our understanding of their needs and offer them a life of wholeness, love, and vitality. Together, let us embark on this journey of holistic pet care, celebrating the intricate and beautiful beings our pets truly are.

Using holistic natural herbs and spices in pet care can offer a multitude of benefits, enhancing the quality of life for our beloved animals in ways that traditional pharmaceutical medicine may not fully achieve. Embracing these time-tested remedies and gentle healing practices can create a harmonious and nurturing approach to pet wellness.

1. Natural and Non-Toxic:
Holistic herbs and spices are derived from nature, making them a safer and non-toxic alternative to many conventional medications. They often have fewer side effects, reducing the risk of adverse reactions and providing gentle relief for various ailments.

2. Whole-Body Healing:

Holistic herbs and spices approach pet care holistically, addressing the underlying causes of issues rather than just treating symptoms. This comprehensive approach supports whole-body healing, promoting overall health and well-being.

3. Individualized Treatment:
Herbal remedies can be tailored to suit the specific needs of each pet. Since animals are unique in their constitution and health requirements, these personalized treatments can offer targeted support for their specific conditions.

4. Natural Immune Support:
Many herbs and spices possess immune-boosting properties, helping to strengthen your pet's immune system and increase their resistance to illnesses. By supporting their immune function, pets can better defend against infections and maintain optimal health.

5. Reduced Dependency on Pharmaceuticals:
Integrating holistic remedies can reduce the reliance on pharmaceutical medications, which are often associated with side effects and long-term health concerns. Using natural alternatives can minimize the need for medications and their potential risks.

6. Improved Digestion:
Certain herbs and spices aid in digestion, supporting optimal gut health in pets. A healthy digestive system contributes to better nutrient absorption, which is essential for overall vitality and energy.

7. Stress and Anxiety Relief:
Herbal remedies are known for their calming effects, helping to reduce stress and anxiety in pets. They can be particularly beneficial during stressful situations such as travel, visits to the vet, or changes in the household.

8. Joint and Mobility Support:
Some herbs and spices possess anti-inflammatory properties, providing relief for joint pain and supporting mobility in aging or arthritic pets. Enhancing their comfort level contributes to a better quality of life.

9. Respiratory Health:
Herbal remedies can help promote healthy respiratory function and alleviate respiratory issues in pets. This is especially beneficial for animals prone to allergies or respiratory conditions.

10. Positive Impact on Behavior:
Certain herbs and spices have a calming effect on behavior, helping to reduce hyperactivity and promote relaxation. This can be particularly useful for pets with behavioral issues or separation anxiety.

By incorporating holistic natural herbs and spices into pet care, we can tap into the wisdom of nature and provide gentle, yet effective, support for our pets' well-being. Embracing these natural remedies fosters a sense of balance and harmony, encouraging a higher quality of life for our furry companions. As responsible pet owners, exploring these natural alternatives can enrich the bond we share with our pets and help them lead a fulfilling and joyful life.

Natural herbs can play a significant role in addressing the emotional well-being of dogs, helping them navigate through various emotional challenges and promoting a balanced and contented state of mind. Here are some examples of natural herbs that have been backed by research and are known for their beneficial effects on dogs' emotional aspect:

1. Chamomile (Matricaria chamomilla):
Chamomile is renowned for its calming properties and is often used to reduce anxiety and stress in dogs. It can help soothe nervousness during stressful situations such as thunderstorms, travel, or visits to the vet. Chamomile's gentle nature makes it a suitable option for promoting relaxation and emotional balance.

2. Valerian Root (Valeriana officinalis):
Valerian root is a potent herb that has been found to have sedative effects on dogs. It can help alleviate anxiety and promote a sense of calmness. Valerian root is often used to support dogs during times of high stress or intense emotional responses.

3. Lavender (Lavandula angustifolia):
Lavender is well-known for its soothing scent, which can help reduce stress and anxiety in dogs. Research has shown that lavender essential oil can have a calming effect, making it a popular choice in aromatherapy for pets.

4. Passionflower (Passiflora incarnata):
Passionflower is another herb with calming properties, beneficial for dogs experiencing anxiety or restlessness. It can help promote relaxation and improve sleep quality, contributing to a sense of emotional well-being.

5. Lemon Balm (Melissa officinalis):
Lemon balm is a gentle herb that has mild sedative effects on dogs. It can help reduce anxiety and nervousness, making it a valuable option for managing emotional stressors.

6. Ashwagandha (Withania somnifera):
Ashwagandha is an adaptogenic herb known for its stress-reducing properties. It helps the body and mind adapt to stress and can be beneficial for dogs experiencing chronic stress or anxiety.

7. Skullcap (Scutellaria lateriflora):
   Skullcap is a calming herb that supports relaxation and emotional stability in dogs. It can be particularly helpful for dogs with hyperactivity or heightened sensitivity to stimuli.

8. St. John's Wort (Hypericum perforatum):
St. John's Wort is a herb that has been traditionally used to support emotional balance in dogs. It may help alleviate mild to moderate anxiety and promote a positive mood.

9. Holy Basil (Ocimum sanctum):
Holy basil is an adaptogenic herb that helps dogs cope with stress and promote emotional resilience. It may also have antioxidant properties, supporting overall well-being.

10. Oatstraw (Avena sativa):
Oatstraw is a gentle nerve tonic that can help soothe and relax dogs experiencing nervousness or anxiety. It provides a nourishing and calming effect on the nervous system.

When considering using herbs for your dog's emotional well-being, it is essential to consult with a veterinarian or a holistic pet care specialist to ensure the appropriate dosage and safety for your pet's specific needs. Incorporating these natural herbs into your dog's daily routine can offer valuable support for their emotional health, leading to a more contented and emotionally balanced life.

Natural herbs can be beneficial in addressing the emotional well-being of cats, providing gentle support to help them cope with various emotional challenges and promoting a sense of tranquility and balance. Here are some examples of natural herbs that have been backed by research and are known for their beneficial effects on cats' emotional aspect:

1. Valerian Root (Valeriana officinalis):
   Valerian root is known for its calming properties and is often used to reduce anxiety and stress in cats. It can help soothe nervousness and promote relaxation, making it a valuable option during times of stress or changes in the environment.

2. Chamomile (Matricaria chamomilla):
   Chamomile is a gentle herb that can help ease anxiety and promote a sense of calmness in cats. It may be beneficial for cats experiencing nervousness or restlessness.

3. Catnip (Nepeta cataria):
Catnip is a well-known herb that has a stimulating effect on cats, inducing feelings of excitement and playfulness. It can also have a calming effect in some cats, helping to reduce stress and anxiety.

4. Lemon Balm (Melissa officinalis):
Lemon balm is a soothing herb that may help calm and relax cats experiencing anxiety or nervousness. It can be useful during stressful situations or transitions.

5. Passionflower (Passiflora incarnata):
Passionflower is an herb known for its calming properties. It can help reduce anxiety and promote relaxation in cats, especially during periods of heightened stress.

6. Skullcap (Scutellaria lateriflora):
   Skullcap is a calming herb that may be beneficial for cats with anxiety or hyperactivity. It can help promote relaxation and emotional stability.

7. Lavender (Lavandula angustifolia):
   Lavender is well-known for its soothing scent, which can have a calming effect on cats. It may help reduce stress and promote a sense of tranquility.

8. Cat's Claw (Uncaria tomentosa):
   Cat's Claw is an adaptogenic herb that can help cats adapt to stress and support their overall emotional well-being.

9. Holy Basil (Ocimum sanctum):
   Holy basil is an adaptogenic herb that may help cats cope with stress and promote emotional resilience.

10. Ashwagandha (Withania somnifera):
    Ashwagandha is an adaptogenic herb that can help cats manage stress and promote a sense of balance and calmness.

As with any herbal remedies, it is essential to consult with a veterinarian or a holistic pet care specialist before using herbs for your cat's emotional well-being. Each cat is unique, and their response to herbs may vary, so it's crucial to determine the appropriate dosage and safety for your pet. By incorporating these natural herbs into your cat's environment or daily routine, you can provide valuable support for their emotional health, contributing to a more serene and contented life.

Chapter 3: The Role of Lifestyle in Pet Health

Our pets' well-being is intricately linked to the lifestyle choices we make for them. Just as our own lifestyle impacts our health and happiness, the same holds true for our beloved animal companions. In this chapter, we explore the profound influence of lifestyle on pets' health and how incorporating holistic practices into their daily lives can lead to a better quality of life and potentially extend their years of joy and vitality.

1. The Connection Between Lifestyle and Pet Health:
   Just like humans, pets thrive in an environment that prioritizes their physical, emotional, and spiritual needs. A balanced lifestyle that includes proper nutrition, regular exercise, mental stimulation, and emotional support is essential for their overall well-being. Engaging in positive and nurturing interactions with our pets fosters a deep bond and contributes to their emotional stability.

2. Nutrition and Wellness:
   Proper nutrition plays a crucial role in pet health, promoting optimal growth, development, and longevity. A well-balanced diet tailored to their individual needs ensures they receive essential nutrients to support their overall vitality and immune system. Embracing natural and whole food options, free from harmful additives, supports their digestive health and reduces the risk of health issues related to poor nutrition.

3. Regular Exercise for Physical and Mental Health:
   Regular exercise is not only essential for maintaining a healthy weight but also for promoting cardiovascular health and joint mobility. Engaging in play and physical activities stimulates their minds, reduces stress, and enhances their overall happiness. Exercise provides a natural outlet for their energy, reducing the risk of behavioral issues that may arise from boredom or inactivity.

4. Holistic Practices for Emotional Balance:
Incorporating holistic practices, such as aromatherapy, herbal remedies, and relaxation techniques, can significantly impact pets' emotional well-being. These practices help reduce stress, anxiety, and fear, promoting emotional stability and resilience. Creating a peaceful and harmonious environment for our pets contributes to their emotional contentment and overall happiness.

5. Creating a Safe and Nurturing Home Environment:
   A safe and nurturing home environment is essential for pets' health and happiness. Minimizing exposure to toxins, providing a comfortable resting place, and ensuring they have a quiet retreat space helps reduce stress and anxiety. A clutter-free and organized living space allows them to move freely and enhances their sense of security.

6. Regular Veterinary Check-ups and Preventive Care:
   Part of a holistic lifestyle for pets includes regular veterinary check-ups and preventive care. Routine health examinations help detect any potential health issues early on, enabling timely

intervention and treatment. Preventive measures, such as vaccinations and parasite control, are essential for safeguarding their health.

7. The Power of Love and Companionship:

Above all, the love, attention, and companionship we offer our pets play a central role in their well-being. Spending quality time with them, engaging in play, and demonstrating affection fosters a strong bond and creates a sense of security and trust. Pets thrive in an environment where they feel cherished and valued as part of the family.

By embracing a holistic lifestyle that integrates natural and nurturing practices, we can provide our pets with the foundation they need for a better quality of life and the potential for extended years of joy and vitality. Our commitment to their overall well-being helps ensure that our cherished companions experience a life filled with love, health, and happiness. As we continue to explore holistic pet care practices, let us celebrate the profound impact our lifestyle choices can have on the lives of our beloved furry friends.

A balanced and enriching lifestyle is the cornerstone of our pets' well-being, offering a multitude of benefits that contribute to their overall health, happiness, and longevity. Just like us, pets thrive when their physical, emotional, and spiritual needs are fulfilled. Here are some key benefits of providing a balanced and enriching lifestyle for our furry companions:

1. Enhanced Physical Health:

A balanced lifestyle that includes regular exercise and a nutritious diet supports pets' physical health and vitality. Physical activities help maintain a healthy weight, strengthen muscles, and improve cardiovascular health. Providing a well-balanced diet with essential nutrients ensures their bodies receive the nourishment they need for optimal function and immune support.

2. Emotional Stability:

Enriching our pets' lives with positive interactions, mental stimulation, and emotional support promotes emotional stability and reduces stress and anxiety. Engaging in play and spending quality time with our pets nurtures their emotional well-being, leading to a happier and more contented state of mind.

3. Improved Behavioral Outcomes:

An enriching lifestyle helps prevent behavioral issues that may arise from boredom or lack of mental stimulation. Providing toys, puzzles, and interactive games engages their minds and curtails destructive behaviors. A balanced lifestyle contributes to well-behaved and well-adjusted pets.

4. Strengthened Bond with Humans:

Interacting with our pets in a positive and nurturing manner fosters a deep bond and a sense of trust between humans and animals. This strong connection enhances communication and understanding, allowing us to better cater to their needs and provide the best care possible.

5. Enhanced Cognitive Function:
Mental stimulation and learning opportunities in their daily lives improve pets' cognitive function and memory retention. Training exercises, new experiences, and problem-solving activities stimulate their minds and keep them engaged and curious.

6. Reduced Risk of Health Issues:
A balanced lifestyle that includes preventive care, regular veterinary check-ups, and a nutritious diet can reduce the risk of various health issues in pets. Early detection of potential health concerns enables timely intervention and treatment, leading to better outcomes.

7. Greater Resilience to Change:
An enriching lifestyle instills a sense of security and resilience in pets, helping them adapt better to changes in their environment or routine. When pets feel comfortable and supported, they are better equipped to handle transitions or new experiences.

8. Increased Lifespan and Quality of Life:
The combination of physical, emotional, and mental enrichment in a balanced lifestyle can potentially extend pets' lifespan and enhance their overall quality of life. A happier and healthier pet is more likely to lead a longer and more fulfilled life.

As responsible pet owners, embracing a balanced and enriching lifestyle for our pets is a rewarding and fulfilling endeavor. By catering to their physical, emotional, and spiritual needs, we create an environment where our beloved companions can flourish, thrive, and share many joyous moments with us. The benefits of a balanced and enriching lifestyle go beyond their individual well-being; they enrich our lives as well, deepening the bond and love we share with our cherished animal companions.

The environment in which our pets live plays a significant role in shaping their health and well-being. From the air they breathe to the spaces they inhabit, the environment has a profound influence on their physical and emotional health. Understanding and optimizing their surroundings can lead to a happier, healthier, and more vibrant life for our beloved animal companions.

1. Air Quality:
Indoor air quality is essential for pets, especially those spending most of their time indoors. Common indoor pollutants like dust, mold, and pet dander can trigger respiratory issues and

allergies. Using air purifiers or ensuring proper ventilation helps maintain clean and fresh air for pets to breathe freely. Avoiding smoking indoors and using pet-safe cleaning products further contributes to a healthier living environment.

2. Temperature and Climate:
Extreme temperatures can have adverse effects on pets' health. In hot weather, pets are susceptible to heatstroke, dehydration, and burned paw pads. Providing ample access to fresh water, shaded areas, and avoiding strenuous outdoor activities during peak heat hours helps protect them from heat-related illnesses. Similarly, during cold weather, ensuring access to warm shelter and cozy bedding helps prevent hypothermia and frostbite.

3. Safety and Hazards:
Identifying and removing potential hazards from the environment is crucial. Toxic plants, chemicals, electrical cords, and small objects that can be ingested pose risks to pets' safety. Pet-proofing living spaces, using childproof latches on cabinets, and keeping harmful substances out of reach safeguard pets from accidents and poisoning.

4. Access to Nature:
Exposure to nature offers numerous benefits to pets' physical and mental health. Regular outdoor walks, playtime in the yard, or exploring nature trails allow pets to engage their senses and experience novel stimuli. Sunlight exposure supports vitamin D synthesis, promoting healthy bones and immune function. Time spent outdoors also reduces the risk of obesity and improves overall fitness.

5. Enrichment and Play:
An enriched environment encourages mental stimulation and physical activity. Providing a variety of toys, puzzles, and interactive games keeps pets engaged and prevents boredom-related behavior, such as excessive barking or destructive chewing. Enrichment activities mimic natural instincts, such as foraging for food or hunting, enhancing pets' overall well-being.

6. Social Interaction:
Socialization is vital for pets' emotional health. Regular interactions with their human family members and other pets foster a sense of belonging and reduce feelings of isolation. Organizing playdates or visits to dog parks allows pets to interact with others, promoting positive social behaviors.

7. Noise and Calmness:
Pets can be sensitive to loud noises and chaotic environments. Loud sounds, such as fireworks or thunderstorms, can trigger anxiety and fear in pets. Creating a designated quiet space or using white noise machines helps reduce stress and provides a safe retreat during stressful events.

8. Routine and Predictability:

Establishing a consistent daily routine brings stability and predictability to pets' lives. Regular feeding times, walks, play sessions, and sleep schedules create a sense of security. Predictability in their routine helps reduce anxiety and increases their sense of trust in their environment.

By addressing these environmental factors, pet owners can create an optimal living space that promotes their pets' health and well-being. A well-balanced environment ensures that pets receive the physical, emotional, and mental support necessary for a fulfilling and happy life. Taking a proactive approach to the environment allows us to be proactive in preventing health issues and providing the best care for our furry companions.

Chapter 4: Promoting Overall Health in Pets

As we delve deeper into the world of pet care, we uncover the significance of a holistic approach in promoting the well-being of our beloved furry companions. Adopting a proactive and preventative mindset is key to ensuring the optimal health and happiness of our pets. In this chapter, we explore the importance of holistic preventative care and the integration of conventional and holistic methods to achieve the best possible outcomes for our pets' overall health.

1. Holistic Preventative Care:
    Taking a holistic approach to preventative care means addressing the physical, emotional, and spiritual needs of our pets before health issues arise. Regular veterinary check-ups, vaccinations, and preventive measures form the foundation of their health. However, we also look beyond the traditional methods and focus on providing a balanced diet, mental stimulation, and emotional support to build resilience and promote wellness.

2. Benefits of Holistic Preventative Care:
Holistic preventative care sets the stage for a healthier and happier life for our pets. By proactively supporting their immune system and overall well-being, we reduce the risk of chronic illnesses and improve their quality of life. A holistic approach also allows us to identify subtle changes in their behavior or health early on, enabling timely intervention and treatment.

3. Integrating Conventional and Holistic Methods:
Embracing both conventional and holistic methods can offer a comprehensive and well-rounded approach to pet care. While conventional medicine provides valuable diagnostic tools and treatments, holistic practices complement these approaches by addressing the root causes of health issues. Integrating the two allows us to provide the best of both worlds, creating an optimal path to wellness.

4. DIY Home Remedies for Pets:

In the upcoming sections, we will share some wonderful DIY home remedies that are safe, natural, and effective for treating common ailments in dogs and cats. These remedies have been carefully curated, backed by research, and can be made easily at home. By utilizing these remedies, pet owners can play a proactive role in their pets' health and well-being.

5. Crafty Comeups and More:

As we journey through this book, we invite you to explore the offerings of Crafty Comeups and More. You can visit craftycomeupsandmore.bigcartel.com to discover a range of holistic pet care products that your pets will adore. Whether you prefer to create your own remedies or opt for ready-made solutions, we have something special in store for every pet owner.

By embracing a holistic approach to pet care and integrating the best of conventional and natural methods, we pave the way for our pets' optimal health and longevity. As you continue reading, you'll uncover a treasure trove of DIY home remedies that will empower you to provide loving and effective care for your furry companions. So, let's embark on this journey together, and let the holistic path guide us towards a world of wellness for our pets.

DIY Homemade Paw Salve Recipe for Itchy Paws (Safe for Dogs and Cats):

Ingredients:
- Coconut oil: Moisturizes and soothes dry and itchy paws. It contains medium-chain fatty acids that promote hydration and nourishment of the paw pads for both dogs and cats.
- Shea butter: Provides additional moisture to dry paws and helps to alleviate itching. Shea butter is rich in vitamins A and E, which have antioxidant properties that support skin health, making it safe for both dogs and cats.
- Beeswax: Creates a protective barrier on the paw pads, shielding them from irritants while locking in moisture. Beeswax is a natural emollient that aids in softening and protecting the skin of both dogs and cats.
- Lavender essential oil: Offers anti-inflammatory properties and helps to soothe and calm irritated paws for both dogs and cats. It also provides a pleasant aroma.
- Chamomile essential oil: Acts as an anti-itch agent and reduces inflammation in the paws of both dogs and cats. Chamomile oil is gentle and calming to the skin of both pets.

Instructions:

Step 1: Gather the Ingredients
- In a clean and dry workspace, gather the coconut oil, shea butter, beeswax, lavender essential oil, and chamomile essential oil. Ensure that all ingredients are of high quality and suitable for topical use on both dogs and cats.

Step 2: Prepare a Double Boiler

- Fill a saucepan with a few inches of water and place it on the stove over medium heat. Set a heat-resistant glass or metal bowl on top of the saucepan, creating a double boiler. The indirect heat will help melt the ingredients gently without overheating them.

Step 3: Melt the Ingredients
- Add 2 tablespoons of coconut oil, 1 tablespoon of shea butter, and 1 tablespoon of beeswax to the double boiler. Stir occasionally with a heat-resistant spoon until all the ingredients are completely melted and blended together.

Step 4: Add Essential Oils
- Remove the double boiler from heat and allow it to cool slightly. Then, add 5-10 drops of lavender essential oil and 5-10 drops of chamomile essential oil to the mixture. Stir well to distribute the oils evenly.

Step 5: Pour into Containers
- Carefully pour the paw salve mixture into small clean containers or tins. You can use empty lip balm containers or small glass jars for this purpose. Leave some space at the top of the containers to avoid spills when closing the lids.

Step 6: Allow to Cool and Solidify
- Let the paw salve containers sit undisturbed at room temperature until they solidify. This may take a few hours. Once solidified, the salve should have a smooth texture and be easy to apply.

Step 7: Application
- To use the paw salve, apply a small amount to your dog's or cat's paws, gently massaging it into the pads and the spaces between the toes. The salve will provide moisturization and soothing relief to their itchy paws.

Note: Always conduct a patch test on a small area of your pet's skin before using the paw salve on a larger area. Discontinue use if any adverse reactions occur. If your pet's paw irritation persists or worsens, consult with a veterinarian for proper diagnosis and treatment.

DIY Homemade Hot Spot Salve Recipe (Safe for Dogs and Cats):

Introduction:
Hot spots, also known as acute moist dermatitis, are common skin irritations that can affect both dogs and cats. These inflamed and painful areas typically appear as red, moist, and sometimes oozy lesions on the skin. Hot spots can cause intense itching, leading pets to lick, chew, or scratch the affected area, exacerbating the irritation. Identifying the causes of hot spots is essential to effectively treating and preventing their occurrence.

Causes of Hotspots in Cats and Dogs:

Hot spots can arise from various factors, often involving underlying skin issues or external triggers. Some common causes of hot spots in both cats and dogs include:

1. Allergies: Allergic reactions to environmental factors, such as pollen, mold, or fleas, can cause intense itching and inflammation, leading to hot spots.

2. Flea Infestations: Flea bites can be highly irritating to pets, and an allergic reaction to flea saliva can trigger hot spots.

3. Poor Grooming: In cats, hot spots can occur due to inadequate grooming, especially in overweight or elderly cats who may have difficulty reaching certain areas.

4. Moisture and Humidity: Dogs that spend a lot of time in wet or humid conditions are more susceptible to hot spots, as moisture can create an ideal environment for bacterial growth.

5. Underlying Skin Conditions: Pets with existing skin issues, such as dermatitis or seborrhea, are more prone to developing hot spots.

DIY Hot Spot Salve Recipe:
To soothe and promote healing in hot spots for both dogs and cats, you can create a natural and safe hot spot salve using the following ingredients:

Ingredients:
- 1/4 cup Coconut oil: Provides moisturization and forms a protective barrier on the affected area, promoting healing and preventing further irritation.
- 1 tablespoon Beeswax: Adds a protective layer to the hot spot, shielding it from external irritants while allowing the skin to breathe.
- 1 tablespoon Shea butter: Offers additional moisture to dry and irritated skin, aiding in the soothing process.
- 1 teaspoon Olive leaf extract: Possesses antibacterial and anti-inflammatory properties, helping to combat infections and reduce redness and swelling.
- 1 teaspoon Calendula infused oil: Soothes and calms irritated skin, supporting the healing process.
- 5-7 drops Lavender essential oil: Offers anti-inflammatory and antimicrobial properties, providing relief and preventing infection.
- 3-5 drops Chamomile essential oil: Acts as an anti-itch agent, reducing the urge to scratch and promoting comfort.

Instructions:

Step 1: Gather the Ingredients
In a clean and dry workspace, gather the coconut oil, beeswax, shea butter, olive leaf extract, calendula infused oil, lavender essential oil, and chamomile essential oil. Ensure that all ingredients are of high quality and suitable for topical use on both dogs and cats.

Step 2: Prepare a Double Boiler
Fill a saucepan with a few inches of water and place it on the stove over medium heat. Set a heat-resistant glass or metal bowl on top of the saucepan, creating a double boiler. The indirect heat will help melt the ingredients gently without overheating them.

Step 3: Melt the Coconut Oil, Beeswax, and Shea Butter
Add 1/4 cup of coconut oil, 1 tablespoon of beeswax, and 1 tablespoon of shea butter to the double boiler. Stir occasionally with a heat-resistant spoon until all the ingredients are completely melted and blended together.

Step 4: Add Olive Leaf Extract and Calendula Infused Oil
Remove the double boiler from heat and allow the melted mixture to cool slightly. Then, add 1 teaspoon of olive leaf extract and 1 teaspoon of calendula infused oil to the mixture. Stir well to combine.

Step 5: Incorporate Essential Oils
Add 5-7 drops of lavender essential oil and 3-5 drops of chamomile essential oil to the mixture. Stir thoroughly to ensure even distribution of the essential oils.

Step 6: Transfer to a Container
Carefully pour the hot spot salve mixture into a clean and shallow container or tin. You can use a small glass jar or any container with a lid that is easy to access when applying the salve.

Step 7: Allow to Cool and Solidify
Let the hot spot salve container sit undisturbed at room temperature until it solidifies. This may take a few hours. Once solidified, the salve should have a smooth texture and be easy to apply.

Step 8: Application
Gently clean the hot spot area on your dog or cat with mild soap and water. Pat dry with a clean towel. Apply a small amount of the salve to the affected area, using clean fingers or a cotton swab. Massage the salve into the hot spot, ensuring even coverage.

Step 9: Repeat as Needed
Apply the hot spot salve 2-3 times a day or as needed to promote healing and provide relief. Continue the application until the hot spot improves and discomfort is alleviated.

Note: Always conduct a patch test on a small area of your pet's skin before using the hot spot salve on a larger area. Discontinue use if any adverse reactions occur. If the hot spot persists or worsens, consult with a veterinarian for proper diagnosis and treatment. Regularly inspect your pet's skin and address any underlying causes to prevent future hot spots.

DIY Homemade Eye Drop Recipe for Eye Infections (Safe for Dogs and Cats):

Introduction:
Eye infections can be a common concern for both dogs and cats, leading to symptoms such as redness, discharge, swelling, and excessive tearing. Proper care and treatment are essential to alleviate discomfort and promote healing. This DIY eye drop recipe contains all-natural, safe, and non-toxic ingredients that can help soothe and cleanse the eyes of your beloved pets.

What is an Eye Infection?
An eye infection in pets is typically caused by bacteria, viruses, allergens, or foreign particles entering the eye and leading to inflammation and irritation. It can affect one or both eyes and may cause discomfort, sensitivity to light, and excessive blinking.

Causes of Eye Infections in Pets:
Several factors can contribute to eye infections in cats and dogs, including:

1. Allergies: Environmental allergens, such as pollen or dust, can cause eye irritation and infections.

2. Bacterial or Viral Infections: Bacteria and viruses can enter the eyes and lead to infections.

3. Foreign Objects: Particles or debris that enter the eyes can cause irritation and lead to infections.

4. Tear Duct Blockage: Blockage in the tear ducts can prevent proper drainage and lead to infections.

DIY Eye Drop Recipe:
To create a natural and safe eye drop solution to treat eye infections in both dogs and cats, you will need the following ingredients:

Ingredients:
- 1/2 cup distilled or boiled and cooled water: Acts as a gentle and sterile base for the eye drops, cleansing and hydrating the eyes.
- 1 teaspoon chamomile tea: Offers soothing properties and helps reduce inflammation and redness in the eyes.
- 1 teaspoon calendula infused oil: Provides antimicrobial and anti-inflammatory benefits, aiding in healing the eye infection.
- 1 drop colloidal silver: Possesses natural antibacterial properties, assisting in combating bacteria in the eyes.
- 1 drop witch hazel extract: Acts as an astringent to help cleanse the eyes and reduce inflammation.
- 1 drop of saline solution (0.9% sodium chloride): Provides an isotonic solution that helps rinse the eyes and flush out debris.

Instructions:

Step 1: Gather the Ingredients
In a clean and dry workspace, gather all the ingredients needed, ensuring they are of high quality and suitable for topical use on both dogs and cats.

Step 2: Prepare the Chamomile Tea
Steep a chamomile tea bag in a small amount of hot water (approximately 1/4 cup) for 5-10 minutes. Allow the tea to cool completely before using it in the eye drop recipe.

Step 3: Mix the Ingredients
In a clean and sterile eye dropper bottle or small glass container with a tight-fitting lid, combine the cooled chamomile tea, distilled or boiled water, calendula infused oil, colloidal silver, witch hazel extract, and saline solution.

Step 4: Shake Well
Gently shake the eye drop solution to ensure all the ingredients are thoroughly combined.

Step 5: Cleanse the Eyes
Before applying the eye drops, gently cleanse your pet's eyes with a damp, clean cloth or a cotton ball soaked in lukewarm water. Gently wipe away any discharge or debris from the corners of the eyes.

Step 6: Administer the Eye Drops
Hold your pet gently but securely, tilting their head slightly upward. Using the eye dropper, carefully instill 1-2 drops of the solution into the corner of the eye. Be sure to aim for the inner corner, as this will allow the solution to spread across the eye effectively.

Step 7: Blinking and Absorption
Allow your pet to blink naturally to distribute the solution across the eye. Repeat the process in the other eye if necessary.

Step 8: Store Properly
Store any remaining eye drop solution in the refrigerator. Before using the solution again, gently warm it to room temperature by holding the bottle between your hands.

Note: If your pet's eye infection persists or worsens, or if there are signs of pain or discomfort, consult with a veterinarian for a thorough examination and appropriate treatment. Proper eye care is crucial to maintain your pet's visual health, and regular check-ups with a veterinarian can help address any eye health concerns promptly.

DIY Home Remedy for Yeast Ear and Skin Infections (liquid form)) (Safe for Dogs and Cats):

Introduction:
Yeast infections in the ears and on the skin can cause discomfort and irritation for both dogs and cats. This DIY home remedy uses all-natural and safe ingredients that can help combat yeast overgrowth and soothe the affected areas, providing relief for your pets.

What is a Yeast Infection?
Yeast infections, also known as fungal infections, in pets occur when there is an overgrowth of yeast organisms on the skin or in the ears. The most common yeast species affecting dogs and cats is Malassezia, which naturally resides on the skin and ears in small amounts. However, factors that disrupt the skin's balance can lead to an overgrowth of these fungi, resulting in an infection.

Causes of Yeast Infections in Dogs and Cats:
Several factors can contribute to yeast infections in dogs and cats, including:

1. Moisture and Warmth: Yeast thrives in warm and moist environments, making areas like the ears, skin folds, and paw pads susceptible to infection, especially in humid climates.

2. Allergies: Pets with allergies, whether food allergies or environmental allergies, may be more prone to yeast infections as their immune system reacts to the allergens, leading to inflammation and creating an ideal environment for yeast to grow.

3. Weakened Immune System: A weakened immune system due to illness, stress, or medication can compromise the body's ability to keep yeast growth in check.

4. Poor Grooming: Pets with thick or long coats, or those that struggle with grooming due to age or other factors, may have a higher risk of yeast infections in areas where moisture and debris accumulate.

5. Underlying Skin Conditions: Pre-existing skin conditions like dermatitis or skin folds can trap moisture and allow yeast to thrive.

6. Excessive Use of Antibiotics: Prolonged use of antibiotics can disrupt the natural balance of bacteria on the skin, allowing yeast to overgrow.

DIY Home Remedy for Yeast Ear and Skin Infections:

Ingredients:
- 2 tablespoons organic apple cider vinegar (with the mother): Contains acetic acid, which helps create an unfavorable environment for yeast growth and aids in restoring the skin's natural pH level.

- 2 tablespoons witch hazel extract: Acts as an astringent, reducing inflammation and promoting healing in the affected areas.
- 1 tablespoon colloidal silver: Possesses natural antibacterial and antifungal properties, combating yeast and bacterial overgrowth.
- 1 tablespoon aloe vera gel: Soothes and moisturizes the skin, providing relief from itching and irritation.
- 1 drop tea tree essential oil: Contains antifungal and antimicrobial properties, assisting in controlling yeast infections.
- 1 drop lavender essential oil: Offers anti-inflammatory and calming effects, promoting skin healing and reducing redness.

Instructions:

Step 1: Gather the Ingredients
In a clean and dry workspace, gather all the ingredients needed, ensuring they are of high quality and suitable for topical use on both dogs and cats.

Step 2: Mix the Ingredients
In a small clean bowl or container, combine the organic apple cider vinegar, witch hazel extract, colloidal silver, aloe vera gel, tea tree essential oil, and lavender essential oil. Stir well to ensure all the ingredients are thoroughly combined.

Step 3: Cleanse the Ears and Affected Skin
Before applying the remedy, gently clean your pet's ears and affected skin with a damp, clean cloth or cotton ball soaked in warm water. Gently remove any discharge or debris from the ears and skin.

Step 4: Apply the Remedy
Using a clean cotton ball or a dropper, carefully apply the prepared DIY remedy to the ears and affected skin. For ear infections, gently lift the ear flap and apply a few drops of the solution into the ear canal. For skin infections, apply the remedy directly to the affected areas.

Step 5: Massage and Soothe
Gently massage the base of the ears or the affected skin to help distribute the remedy. This will also help soothe your pet and provide comfort.

Step 6: Allow to Dry
Allow the remedy to air dry on your pet's ears and skin. Avoid touching or rubbing the areas during the drying process.

Step 7: Repeat as Needed
For best results, apply the DIY remedy 2-3 times a day or as directed by your veterinarian, until the yeast infection subsides and the skin shows signs of improvement.

Note: If your pet's condition worsens or if there are signs of discomfort or adverse reactions, discontinue use and consult with a veterinarian for further evaluation and appropriate treatment. While this DIY home remedy is generally safe for most pets, individual sensitivities can vary, and it's always best to seek professional advice when dealing with persistent health issues. Regular check-ups with a veterinarian can also help monitor your pet's overall health and well-being.

DIY Homemade Salve for Ear and Skin Yeast Infections (Safe for Dogs and Cats)

The following recipe is to make a DIY salve.

Ingredients and Their Health Benefits:
- 1/4 cup coconut oil: Provides moisturization and forms a protective barrier on the skin and in the ears, promoting healing and preventing further irritation.
- 1 tablespoon calendula infused oil: Soothes and calms irritated skin and ears, supporting the healing process.
- 1 tablespoon beeswax: Creates a protective layer over the affected areas, shielding them from external irritants while allowing the skin to breathe.
- ⅓ teaspoon of Olive Leaf Extract: Possesses natural antibacterial and antifungal properties, combating yeast and bacterial overgrowth.
- 1 drop tea tree essential oil: Contains antifungal and antimicrobial properties, assisting in controlling yeast infections.
- 1 drop lavender essential oil: Offers anti-inflammatory and calming effects, promoting skin healing and reducing redness.

Instructions:

Step 1: Gather the Ingredients
In a clean and dry workspace, gather all the ingredients needed, ensuring they are of high quality and suitable for topical use on both dogs and cats.

Step 2: Prepare a Double Boiler
Fill a saucepan with a few inches of water and place it on the stove over medium heat. Set a heat-resistant glass or metal bowl on top of the saucepan, creating a double boiler. The indirect heat will help melt the ingredients gently without overheating them.

Step 3: Melt the Coconut Oil and Beeswax
Add 1/4 cup of coconut oil and 1 tablespoon of beeswax to the double boiler. Stir occasionally with a heat-resistant spoon until they are completely melted and blended together.

Step 4: Add Calendula Infused Oil

Remove the double boiler from heat and allow the melted mixture to cool slightly. Then, add 1 tablespoon of calendula infused oil and. Stir well to combine.

Step 5: Incorporate Essential Oils
Add 10 drops of tea tree essential oil, and 10 drop of lavender essential oil to the mixture. Stir thoroughly to ensure even distribution of the ingredients.

Step 6: Transfer to a Container
Carefully pour the salve mixture into a clean and shallow container or tin. You can use a small glass jar or any container with a lid that is easy to access when applying the salve.

Step 7: Allow to Solidify
Let the salve container sit undisturbed at room temperature until it solidifies. This may take a few hours. Once solidified, the salve should have a smooth texture and be easy to apply.

Step 8: Application
For skin infections, gently cleanse the affected area with a damp, clean cloth or cotton ball soaked in warm water. Pat dry with a clean towel. Apply a small amount of the salve to the affected skin and massage it in gently.

For ear infections, using gloves, apply a dime sized amount of the salve to the ear canal, avoiding deep insertion. Gently massage the base of the ear to help distribute the salve.

Step 9: Repeat as Needed
Apply the DIY salve 2-3 times a day or as directed by your veterinarian, until the yeast infection subsides and the skin or ears show signs of improvement.

Note: If your pet's condition worsens or if there are signs of discomfort or adverse reactions, discontinue use and consult with a veterinarian for further evaluation and appropriate treatment. While this DIY salve is generally safe for most pets, individual sensitivities can vary, and it's always best to seek professional advice when dealing with persistent health issues. Regular check-ups with a veterinarian can also help monitor your pet's overall health and well-being.

DIY Homemade Flea and Tick Shampoo (Safe for Dogs and Cats):

Introduction:
Fleas and ticks can be a pesky problem for both dogs and cats, causing discomfort and potential health issues. This DIY shampoo recipe uses all-natural and safe ingredients that can help repel and treat fleas and ticks, providing a gentle yet effective solution for your pets.

Ingredients and Their Health Benefits:
- 1 cup liquid castile soap: Acts as a gentle cleanser, removing dirt and debris from your pet's coat without causing irritation.
- 1 tablespoon neem oil: Possesses natural insect-repelling properties, helping to keep fleas and ticks at bay.
- 1 tablespoon almond oil: Provides moisturization and nourishment to your pet's skin and coat, promoting a healthy and shiny appearance.
- 5-7 drops lavender essential oil: Offers a pleasant scent and contains anti-inflammatory properties, soothing the skin and reducing irritation.
- 1 tablespoon apple cider vinegar: Helps balance the skin's pH level, making it less favorable for fleas and ticks.

Instructions:

Step 1: Gather the Ingredients
In a clean and dry workspace, gather all the ingredients needed, ensuring they are of high quality and suitable for topical use on both dogs and cats.

Step 2: Mix the Ingredients
In a clean and empty shampoo bottle or container, combine the liquid castile soap, neem oil, almond oil, lavender essential oil, and apple cider vinegar. Gently shake or stir the mixture to ensure all the ingredients are thoroughly combined.

Step 3: Wet Your Pet's Coat
Before applying the DIY shampoo, wet your pet's coat thoroughly with warm water. Ensure that the water is not too hot, as it may cause discomfort.

Step 4: Apply the Shampoo
Squeeze a small amount of the DIY flea and tick shampoo into your hand and lather it onto your pet's coat. Start at the neck and work your way down, making sure to cover all areas, including underbelly and legs. Be gentle and avoid getting the shampoo into your pet's eyes and ears.

Step 5: Massage and Soak
Gently massage the shampoo into your pet's coat and skin, ensuring that it reaches the fur's roots. Let the shampoo soak on your pet's coat for a few minutes, allowing the natural ingredients to work their magic.

Step 6: Rinse Thoroughly
Thoroughly rinse your pet's coat with warm water, making sure to remove all traces of the shampoo.

Step 7: Repeat if Necessary
If your pet has a severe flea or tick infestation, you can repeat the shampooing process. However, for regular use, it's best to shampoo your pet once every 1-2 weeks or as needed.

Step 8: Towel Dry
Gently towel dry your pet, removing excess water from their coat. Allow your pet to air dry or use a hairdryer on a low setting if they are comfortable with it.

Note: While this DIY flea and tick shampoo is generally safe for most pets, individual sensitivities can vary. Always conduct a patch test on a small area of your pet's skin before using the shampoo on a larger area. Discontinue use if any adverse reactions occur. If your pet experiences any discomfort or severe flea or tick issues persist, consult with a veterinarian for appropriate treatment and prevention measures. Regularly inspect your pet's coat for fleas and ticks and address any underlying causes to keep them happy and pest-free.

Closing:

Thank you for joining me on this journey through the world of holistic health for our beloved pets. As a passionate advocate for natural remedies and a firm believer in the power of holistic healing, I hope you find the recipes and insights shared in this book valuable in providing a safer and healthier life for your furry companions.

Before we part ways, I must reiterate the important disclaimer that I am not a Doctor or a Veterinarian. While I firmly believe in the benefits of a natural holistic approach for our pets, it is essential to consult your own healthcare provider or veterinarian for any specific health concerns or questions. Your pet's well-being is of utmost importance, and professional guidance is always advisable.

As we conclude this book, I would like to take a moment to introduce my business, Crafty Comeups and More. My name is Bernadette Knight, and through Crafty Comeups and More, I offer a range of creative and customizable products and services. My graphic design capabilities enable me to help you create stunning invitations, business cards, and promotional tools, including eye-catching logos for your businesses.

At Crafty Comeups and More, we take pride in our array of customizable items, from fun and unique T-shirts for bachelorette parties, bachelor parties, and other occasions to stylish clothing and accessories for our beloved dogs and cats. Additionally, we offer a delightful selection of coffee mugs, tote bags, and so much more.

As a token of appreciation for your purchase of this book, I would like to extend a special thank-you gift. By contacting me with a screenshot of your purchase of this book and providing your shipping information, you will receive a free Lotto scratch-off card. This card gives you the chance to win exciting free prizes or services connected to Crafty Comeups and More.

To redeem your free scratch-off card, please visit my website: craftycomeupsandmore.bigcartel.com. I am thrilled to share this little surprise with you as a gesture of gratitude for supporting my passion for holistic health and creative endeavors.

Once again, thank you for choosing this book, and I sincerely hope it brings you and your pets a wealth of benefits and joy. Wishing you and your furry friends a vibrant and healthy life ahead!

As an added bonus, I would like to introduce you to my partnering website, BRIODS.COM. Led by CEO and Director of Business Development, Avidon Respes, BRIODS stands for Boss, Revolutionist, Innovator, Opportunist, Developer, and Strategist. BRIODS is dedicated to empowering individuals like you with exclusive products, exciting investment opportunities, and invaluable knowledge to help you succeed in all your business endeavors.

At BRIODS, you can explore an exquisite collection of exclusive brand apparel, representing the spirit of entrepreneurship and ambition. Additionally, BRIODS offers exciting investment opportunities that can pave the way for your financial growth and prosperity.

But that's not all! BRIODS is committed to empowering you with the skills needed to become a successfulentrepreneur.Throughdynamicclassesandworkshops,youcanlearnessential strategies to gain financial freedom and master the art of succeeding in your business ventures.

To discover more about BRIODS and all the incredible products and services they offer, I invite you to visit their website, BRIODS.COM. Here, you will find a wealth of resources and opportunities that can transform your entrepreneurial journey.

As a gesture of appreciation for your support, I would love to send you a raffle scratch-off lottery card on behalf of BRIODS Corporation of America. This card gives you a chance to win awesome prizes, adding a sprinkle of excitement to your path of success.

To receive your raffle scratch-off card, please contact me with a screenshot of your purchase of this book, along with your shipping information. It is my sincere wish that this surprise brings you joy and further enriches your journey toward holistic health and business prosperity.

I would like to give a special shout-out to Avidon Respes, the CEO and Director of Business Development at BRIODS.COM. Avidon, I am incredibly grateful to you for giving me the opportunity to work closely with you and for being an invaluable mentor in my journey as an entrepreneur. Your guidance and support have helped me grow my business, Crafty Comeups and More, and become more versatile in my capabilities.

Thank you, Avidon, for sharing your expertise and teaching me everything I needed to know to be successful in this industry. Your belief in me and your encouragement to explore my creativity have allowed me to create amazing and unique products for my customers.

Most importantly, I want to express my gratitude for the life lessons you've imparted. You've shown me the importance of believing in myself and my ideas, as well as the value of hard work and dedication to my craft. Your mentorship has been invaluable, and I am truly honored to have you as a guiding force in my entrepreneurial journey.

To all the readers, I invite you to explore the incredible opportunities that BRIODS.COM has to offer. From exclusive brand apparel to exciting investment ventures and empowering classes, Avidon and the team at BRIODS are dedicated to supporting your path to success.

And don't forget, you can also find some of my handmade holistic pet care products on my website, craftycomeupsandmore.bigcartel.com. These products have been crafted with love and care, using natural and safe ingredients to promote the well-being of your furry companions.

As a token of appreciation for your support, I would love to send you a raffle scratch-off lottery card on behalf of BRIODS Corporation of America. This card gives you a chance to win awesome prizes, adding a sprinkle of excitement to your path of success.

To receive your raffle scratch-off card, please contact me with a screenshot of your purchase of this book, along with your shipping information. It is my sincere wish that this surprise brings you joy and further enriches your journey toward holistic health and business prosperity.

Thank you once again for choosing this book, and I sincerely hope it brings you and your pets a wealth of benefits and joy. Wishing you and your furry friends a vibrant and healthy life ahead!

With warm regards,

Bernadette Knight
Crafty Comeups and More

I SPECIALIZE IN A VARIETY
OF THINGS SUCH AS:

GRAPHIC DESIGN

I CAN HELP YOU CREATE INVITATIONS ,
BUSINESS CARDS, AND PROMOTIONAL
TOOLS AND LOGOS FOR BUSINESSES;
JUST TO NAME A FEW.

CUSTOMIZABLE ITEMS

T-SHIRTS FOR BACHELORETTE
PARTIES , BACHELOR PARTIES,
FUNERALS, BABY SHOWERS ETC..
DOG AND CAT CLOTHING AND
ACCESSORIES, COFFEE MUGS, TOTE
BAGS AND MORE.

Make sure you visit
my partnering
website
BRIODS.com
for help with starting
your own business or
growing your current
business , exciting
investment
opportunities and so
much more.

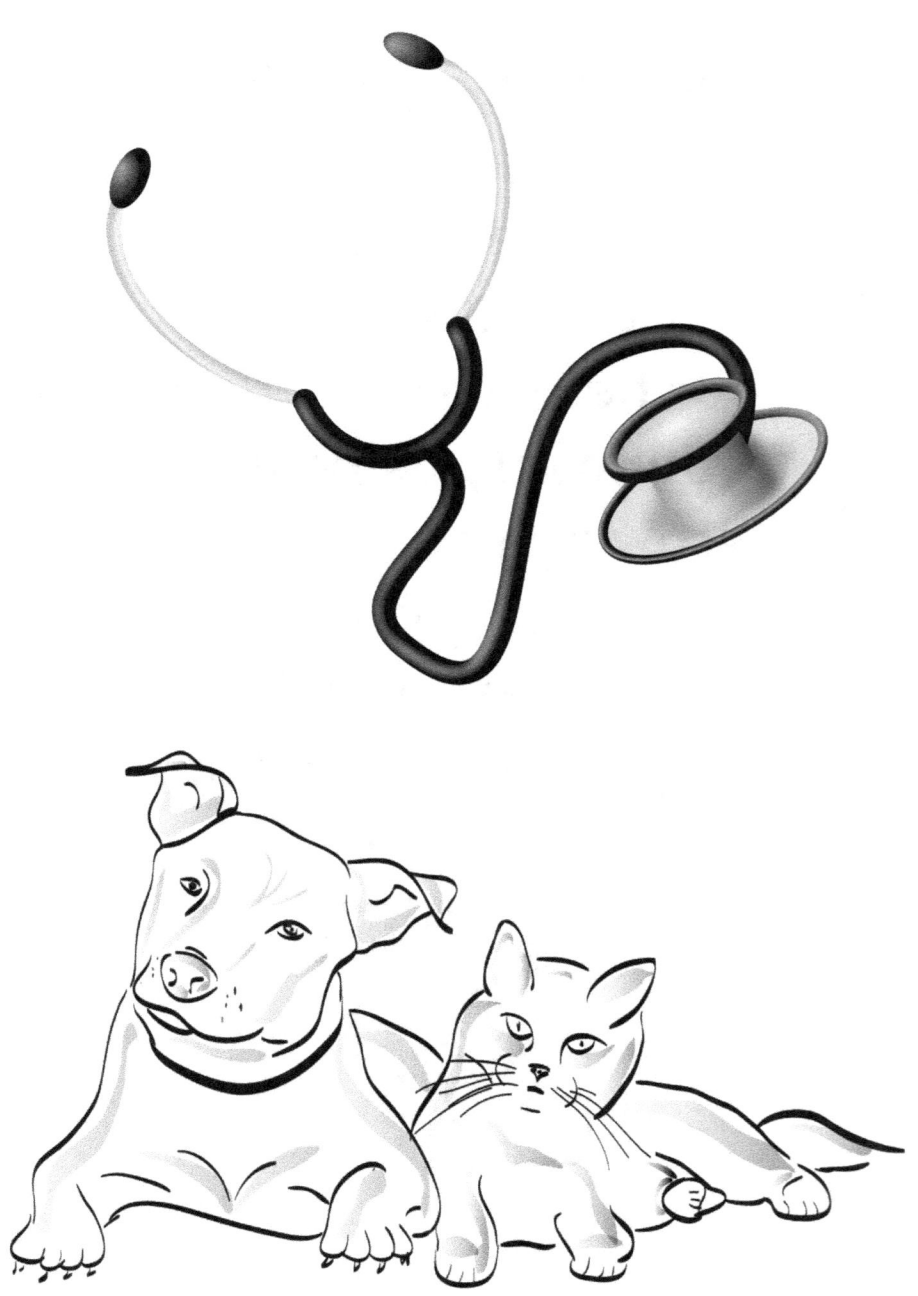